DK Natural Care Library
DONG QUAI
WOMAN'S WONDER DRUG

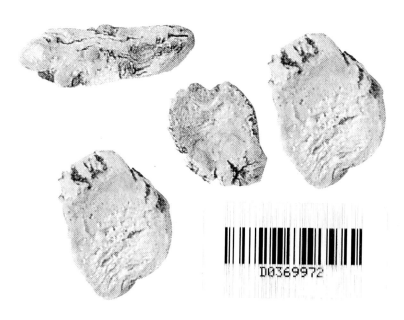

By STEPHANIE PEDERSEN

DORLING KINDERSLEY PUBLISHING, INC.
www.dk.com

CONTENTS

HERBAL HISTORY

Long before over-the-counter medications and prescription drugs came on the scene, herbs proved to be powerful healers. Every culture on earth has used herbal medicine. In fact, herbal usage is older than recorded history itself: Herbal preparations were found in the burial site of a Neanderthal man who lived over 60,000 years ago.

When it comes to herbal medicine, many healing systems are available and useful. Perhaps the best known are ayurveda, Chinese medicine, and Western herbalism. Ayurveda is a system of diagnosis and treatment that uses herbs in conjunction with breathing, meditation, and yoga. It has been practiced in India for more than 2,500 years. Ayurveda gets its name from the Sanskrit words *ayuh*, meaning "longevity," and *veda*, meaning "knowledge." Indeed, in ayurvedic healing, health can be achieved only after identifying a person's physical and mental characteristics (called *dosha*). Then the proper preventative or therapeutic remedies are prescribed to help an individual maintain doshic balance.

Chinese medicine is another healing system that uses herbs, in combination with acupressure, acupuncture, and qi gong. Sometimes called traditional Chinese medicine (TCM), this ancient system is thought to be rooted as far back as 2800 BC in the time of emperor Sheng Nung. Known as China's patron saint of herbal medicine, Sheng Nung is credited among the first proponents of healing plants. Chinese medicine attempts to help the body correct energy imbalances. Therefore herbs are classified according to certain active characteristics, such as heating, cooling, moisturizing, or drying, and prescribed according to how they influence the activity of various organ systems.

Many herbal practitioners believe that Western herbalism can trace its roots to the ancient Sumerians, who—according to a medicinal recipe dating from 3000 BC—boasted a refined knowledge of herbal medicine. Records from subsequent cultures, such as the Assyrians, Egyptians, Israelites, Greeks, and Romans, show similar herbal healing systems. But these peoples weren't the only ones using beneficial plants. The Celts, Gauls, Scandinavians, and other early European tribes also healed with herbs. In fact, it was their knowledge, melded with the medicine brought by invading Moors and Romans, that formed the foundation for Western herbalism. Simply put, this foundation formed a comprehensive system wherein herbs were grouped according to how they affected both the body and specific body systems.

Western herbalism was refined further when Europeans traveled to the New World. Once here, the Europeans fused their medical knowledge with that of the Native Americans. Herbal know-how became an important part of early American habits, so that wellness remedies were handed down from mothers to daughters to granddaughters, and medicinal plants were grown in home gardens. Physicians from the 1600s, 1700s, 1800s, and early 1900s commonly used plants such as arnica, echinacea, and garlic to heal patients. Herbs were listed as medicine in official publications such as the *United States Pharmacopoeia* (the definitive American listing) and the *National Formulary* (the pharmacist's handbook). With the creation of synthetic medications in the 1930s, herbal medicine began to wane.

Fortunately, Europeans and Asians never gave up their herbal remedies. Instead, they used them to complement synthetic medications. Their successes—combined with the desire of many Americans for alternatives to the high price tags and unforgiving side effects of synthetic drugs—have kept the world moving forward on a healthier herbal path.

WHAT IS DONG QUAI?

Dong quai (pronounced "dong-kway") may not have the familiar-sounding ring of some better-known herbs. But the lack of familiarity doesn't make it any less potent. Dong quai is no medicinal newcomer—the herb boasts a long, distinguished history as an analgesic, blood tonic, diuretic, muscle regulator, and sedative. The herb was first mentioned in Chinese herbal literature in the *Collection of Commentaries on the Materia Medica*, dating back to about 500 BC. According to this ancient record, Chinese healers used dong quai both for "female" conditions—such as childbirth, irregular menses, infertility, painful menses, and postpartum pain—and for ailments that affected both sexes, including constipation, stomachaches, and conditions of the circulatory system, heart, liver, and nervous system.

Many Americans and Europeans may be more familiar with a near-cousin of dong quai's, *Angelica archangelica* (commonly called angelica), the essential oils of which are used as an ingredient in cosmetics and a flavoring in the alcoholic drinks Benedictine, chartreuse, and gin. Both herbs have similar therapeutic properties, but dong quai (which is native to the East) is a far more potent blood tonic than is angelica (which is native to the West). The German Commission E monographs also list dong quai as a treatment for gastrointestinal relief. Furthermore, the herb is frequently prescribed throughout Europe (and by some American physicians) for heartburn, flatulence, and as a menopausal aid.

Indeed, it is as a menopausal aid that dong quai has caught the public's attention. Research has shown that dong quai produces a balancing effect on estrogen, helping to relieve symptoms of menopause such as vaginal dryness and headaches. The herb also contains phytoestrogens, or plant estrogens. Phytoestrogens have been shown to help relieve hot flashes.

Dong quai's therapeutic actions, however, go beyond being only a menopausal helper. Researchers studying the herb have isolated at least six coumarin derivatives that exert antispasmodic and vasodilatory effects. The essential oil in dong quai contains ligustilide, butylphalide, and numerous other minor components. Ferulic acid and various polysaccharides are also found in dong quai's root. These elements can prevent spasms, reduce blood clotting, and relax peripheral blood vessels. Other substances include vitamins E, A, and B_{12}. Dong quai is a fragrant perennial native to China, Japan, and Korea. A member of the Umbelliferae family, it is related to the carrot. Just like its vegetable cousin, it is dong quai's that is used. In China, this root is most often made into tea or eaten as a vegetable—sliced and steamed in wine, chopped and added to soups, or fried with garlic.

IN OTHER WORDS
Like many herbs, dong quai is known by many names. Here are some of them:

* Angelica Root
* Angelica Sinensis
* Angelica Polymorpha
* Chinese Angelica
* Empress of the Herbs
* Female Ginseng
* Dang Gui
* Dong Gui
* Tang Gui
* Tang Kwei

SCIENCE TALK

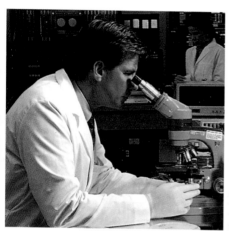

MEDICINE WORLDWIDE
According to an estimate made by the National Institutes of Health, only 10 to 30 percent of the health care worldwide is allopathic, or "Western." The rest of the world's medical care is what Americans would call "alternative," including ayurveda, energy healing, herbalism, homeopathy and traditional Chinese medicine.

CELEBRATING GERMAN KNOW-HOW
Perhaps no other country in the Western world has done more than Germany to further the cause of herbal medicine. What's the country's secret? Commission E, a review board of respected pharmacologists, physicians, and scientists. The board was established in 1978, and members spent the first 15 years researching more than 300 age-old herbs for preparations, usages, recommended dosages, and side effects. Then, in 1980, the German government upped the medical ante, creating a mandate requiring all new herbal remedies sold in pharmacies to meet the same criteria as over-the-counter drugs. To comply, researchers performed thousands of rigorous clinical trials, resulting in a deep well of knowledge used by doctors open to herbs worldwide.

DO YOU HAVE A CONTRAINDICATION?

Before taking any herb, it's important to ask your physician whether you have any contraindications.

What does "contraindication" mean? It's a common medical term that refers to a symptom or condition that makes a particular treatment inadvisable. For example, because dong quai has a documented laxative effect, any illness characterized by diarrhea, such as food poisoning, is a contraindication.

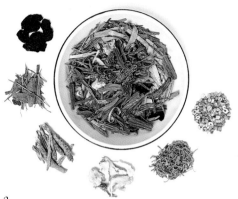

Before taking any herb, ask yourself the following questions:

✔ Have I done any background research on the herb?

✔ What condition am I taking this herb for?

✔ Am I taking other medications or herbs that may affect the herb's functioning?

✔ Do I have any preexisting condition that is contraindicated?

✔ Am I pregnant, trying to conceive, or nursing?

✔ Have I spoken to my physician, a naturopathic doctor, or an herbalist before taking this herb?

✔ Do I know the proper dosages for the herb?

COMMON SIDE EFFECTS

Many medicinal herbs cause mild side effects. Here's what a small number of dong quai users experience:

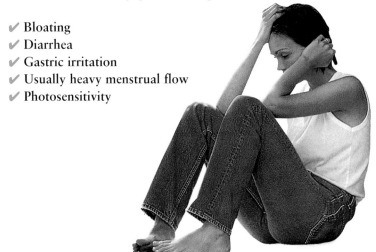

- ✔ Bloating
- ✔ Diarrhea
- ✔ Gastric irritation
- ✔ Usually heavy menstrual flow
- ✔ Photosensitivity

WHAT TO LOOK FOR

In the market for a dong quai remedy, but you're not sure how to choose one? Here's a hint: The most effective remedies boast a high concentration of active ingredients called ligustilides. To ensure that you get the most potent—and beneficial—medicine available, look for products standardized to 1.0 to 1.1 percent ligustilides per 200-mg dose.

PRECAUTIONS

✖ Because dong quai stimulates menstrual flow, it should not be taken by individuals who experience heavy periods.

✖ Although some doctors of Chinese medicine use dong quai to stimulate uterine contractions during childbirth, if you are pregnant, we recommend that you do not use dong quai.

✖ Because dong quai inhibits blood coagulation, do not use it if you have a blood-clotting disorder.

✖ Since dong quai contains estrogen-like chemicals, do not use the herb if you have estrogen-sensitive fibroids or cancer.

✖ Dong quai can cause severe photosensitivity in sun-sensitive individuals.

✖ Dong quai essential oil should never be taken internally. It contains a potentially carcinogenic substance called safrole.

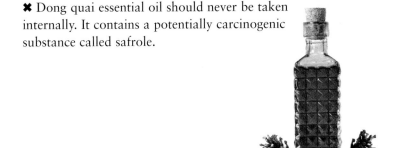

FORMULA GUIDE

Capsules, extracts, teas, tinctures—what do they all mean?
For the uninitiated, we offer this guide to herbal formulas:

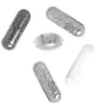

✴ **Capsules.** The medicinal part of the herb is freeze-dried, pulverized, and packed into gelatin capsules. Dong quai capsules usually contain anywhere from 200 mg to 600 mg of herb powder; occasionally the dried herb is reinforced with concentrated extracts.

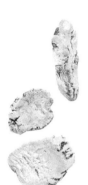

✴ **Herb, Dried.** The flowers, leaves, stems, and/or roots of many herbs are often available dried at health food stores and herbal pharmacies. While these are most commonly made into homemade teas, they can also be used to make decoctions, infused oils, sachets, and more.

✴ **Herb, Fresh.** Herbs that are used in both culinary and medicinal ways (such as dill, garlic, or parsley) are most often found fresh. These can be made into homemade extract, juice, infused oil, tea, and more.

✴ **Juices.** The extracted juice from fresh herbs can be found mixed with commercially prepared fruit or vegetable juices.

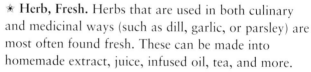

✴ **Liquid Extract** (also called Extract). Macerated plant material is steeped over a period of time in a solvent or solvents such as alcohol, glycerin, and/or water. The steeped liquid is then reduced to lessen the concentration of (or entirely remove) the solvents. Generally stronger than a tincture.

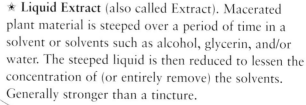

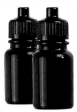

★ **Oil, Essential** (also called Oil). Essential oils are the volatile oily components of herbs. They are found in tiny glands located in the flowers, leaves, roots, and/or bark and are mechanically or chemically extracted. Essential oil is prescribed almost exclusively for external use.

★ **Oil, Infused.** Made by steeping fresh or dried herbs in an edible oil. After a period of time, the herbs are removed and the oil used internally or externally. Not as potent as essential oil.

★ **Ointments.** Dried or fresh herbs are steeped in a base of oils and emulsifiers (such as beeswax, petroleum jelly, or soft paraffin wax). After a period of time, the herbs are removed and the ointment packaged. For external use only.

★ **Syrups.** Syrups are usually a combination of herbal extracts and a sweetener, such as honey or sugar. Generally used for colds, flu, and sore throats.

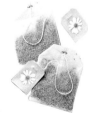

★ **Teas/Infusions.** The words "tea" and "infusion" are often used interchangeably in herbal healing. While commercial herbal tea bags are available, herbal tea can also be made with loose dried or fresh herbs.

★ **Tinctures.** Plant material is soaked in alcohol. The saturated plant material is then pressed. Liquid from this pressing may be diluted with water and packaged—usually in small dropper bottles.

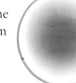

CONDITIONS AND DOSES

CORONARY ARTERY DISEASE

❏ **Symptoms:** Coronary artery disease accounts for about one in two American deaths each year. The disease progresses slowly over the course of years and even decades, but its impact can be instantaneous: In nearly one-third of all cases, death occurs without any previous warning of disease. Indeed, some people have no symptoms, while others may experience chest pain, constriction, or a sense of heaviness in the chest; fatigue; pallor; shortness of breath; swelling in the ankles; and weakness. Coronary artery disease occurs when cholesterol deposits build up on coronary artery walls. These special blood vessels provide oxygen and nutrients to the muscles of the heart. When they are unable to deliver adequate blood flow, however, the heart muscle begins to weaken, leading to angina (chest pain), congestive heart failure, and heart attack. When it comes to causes, a high-fat diet is most often implicated, although heredity, stress, inactivity, smoking, and alcoholism are also culprits.

❏ **How Dong Quai Can Help:** Several studies have shown that dong quai combats coronary artery disease in two ways. The coumarins in dong quai act as a vasodilator, opening up clogged, hardened blood vessels so blood can more easily travel through. The coumarins also keep blood platelets from becoming sticky and thick; thin blood can more easily pass through blocked arteries.

❒ **Dosages:** If you are currently being treated for coronary artery disease, do not take dong quai without first consulting your cardiologist. If given the go-ahead, take one 200-mg capsule three times a day; or 1/4 teaspoon of liquid extract three times a day; or 1/2 teaspoon of tincture three times a day. Dong quai can be taken as a companion to other herbal remedies for coronary artery disease.

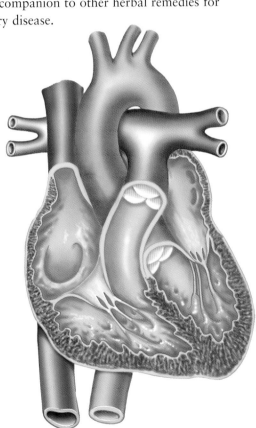

CONDITIONS AND DOSES

HIGH BLOOD CHOLESTEROL

❏ **Symptoms:** High blood cholesterol refers to high levels of fat in the blood. Blame the condition on a fatty diet, heredity, alcoholism, smoking, sedentary lifestyle, or a combination thereof—whatever the cause, the condition is dangerous. Gummy in texture, fat thickens blood and gets stuck on artery walls, thus increasing one's risk of coronary artery disease, heart attack, and stroke. Symptoms can include chest pain, lethargy, pallor, and shortness of breath. However, the condition is often asymptomatic; many individuals learn they have high cholesterol only after a routine blood test.

❏ **How Dong Quai Can Help:** While dong quai does not lower serum cholesterol levels, it is one of many complementary measures that help treat high blood cholesterol. The herb works by thinning fat-thickened blood, helping it pass more easily through blood vessels. Other important steps to lowering serum cholesterol levels include adopting a low-fat, vegetarian or near-vegetarian diet, quitting cigarettes, and exercising regularly.

❏ **Dosages:** If you are currently being treated for high cholesterol, do not take dong quai without first consulting your cardiologist. If given the go-ahead, take one 200-mg capsule, three times a day; or 1/4 teaspoon of liquid extract three times a day; or 1/2 teaspoon of tincture three times a day. Dong quai can be taken as a companion to other cholesterol-lowering herbal remedies.

LIVER LOVER

The liver is the largest single internal organ in the
body, weighing as much as four pounds. It is also one
of the most complex organs, responsible for regulating
the composition of the blood, metabolizing nutrients
that are absorbed from the intestine and converting
these nutrients into forms that can be used by the
body, and detoxifying the blood by removing drugs,
alcohol, and other potentially harmful chemicals from
the bloodstream. Yet exposure to alcohol, chemicals,
or certain viruses can damage the liver and make it
difficult for the organ to perform one or more of its
functions. Fortunately, dong quai can help. Studies
have shown that the herb increases nutrient
metabolism by the liver and helps the liver more
efficiently detoxify the blood.

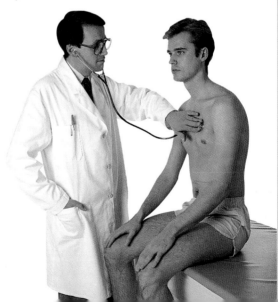

CONDITIONS AND DOSES

HYPERTENSION

❒ **Symptoms:** Hypertension, more commonly known as high blood pressure, is a condition in which blood travels through the arteries at higher-than-normal pressure. This increased blood flow literally wears out the blood vessels, heart, and kidneys and can lead to premature death. What causes hypertension? Cigarettes, alcohol, some medications, and certain illnesses can elevate blood pressure, but by far the most common cause of hypertension is clogged arteries from a high-fat diet. When blood vessels are blocked with fatty deposits, the heart must work harder to move the same amount of blood through them. This in turn increases the pressure at which the blood is pumped. Unfortunately, hypertension is symptomless, leaving many individuals unaware that they even suffer from the condition—until it's too late.

❒ **How Dong Quai Can Help:** Dong quai helps treat hypertension by inhibiting coagulation, so blood doesn't clog on cholesterol deposits as it moves through the veins.

❒ **Dosages:** If you are currently being treated for hypertension, do not take dong quai without first consulting your cardiologist. If given the go-ahead, take one 200-mg capsule three times a day; or 1/4 teaspoon of liquid extract three times a day; or 1/2 teaspoon of tincture three times a day. Dong quai can be taken as a companion to other herbal remedies for hypertension.

A DIABETIC HELPER?

To understand diabetes, it helps to know something about the pancreas. The organ—long and thin and situated behind the stomach—is responsible for regulating the body's use of glucose. To do so, the pancreas creates a number of chemicals, including insulin. When blood glucose levels begin to rise, it is insulin's job to prod muscle and fat cells to absorb whatever glucose they need for future activities; the liver stores any leftover surplus. Yet, some individuals either do not produce enough insulin or their body resists whatever insulin is produced, an outside source is required. Either way, the result is the same: diabetes—diabetes type 1 (juvenile-onset diabetes) and diabetes type 2 (adult-onset diabetes), respectively. Symptoms of both types include blurred vision, fatigue, frequent bladder infections, increased appetite, increased thirst, increased urination, nausea, skin infections, vaginitis, and vomiting. If not treated, diabetes can cause blood vessel damage, gangrene, heart attack, kidney damage, nerve damage, stroke, and vision problems.

Enter dong quai. In Chinese medicine, the herb is used to treat diabetic symptoms. Modern studies have found the herb effective in lowering blood sugar levels. Dong quai has also been shown to help lower the risk of coronary artery disease, a common complication of long-term diabetes. While the herb can be taken safely in tandem with synthetic or other herbal diabetes treatments, it is important to consult your physician before self-medicating with dong quai.

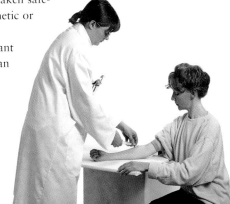

CONDITIONS AND DOSES

CYSTITIS

❏ **Symptoms:** Cystitis is an inflammation of the bladder. Commonly called a bladder infection, the condition is most often caused by escherichia coli, a bacterium that lives in the intestines. Symptoms include cloudy urine (which may contain blood), frequent urination, lower abdominal pain, an urgent desire to empty the bladder, and painful burning during urination

❏ **How Dong Quai Can Help:** Dong quai has long been used in Chinese medicine to treat bladder infections. Indeed, the herb have been shown to combat the escherichia coli bacterium which causes cystitis. In addition, the herb has been shown to promote urination by increasing urine output.

❏ **Dosages:** At the first sign of infection, enjoy 1 or 2 cups of dong quai tea. For stronger relief, take one 200-mg capsule, three times a day; or 1/4 teaspoon of liquid extract three times a day; or 1/2 teaspoon of tincture three times a day.

LOSE THE WATER
In Chinese medicine, dong quai is used
for a variety of ailments, including
water retention. Indeed, the herb has
been shown in studies to exhibit
strong diuretic qualities, thus helping
the body release trapped liquid
through the urinary tract.

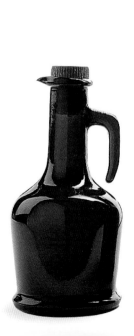
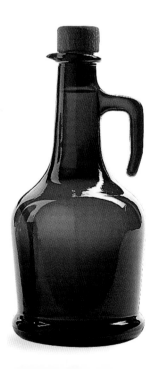

CONDITIONS AND DOSES

FATIGUE

❏ **Symptoms:** Fatigue is a side effect of many medical and nonmedical conditions, including anemia, depression, illness, mental exertion, physical exertion, and stress. Signs of fatigue include mental and physical exhaustion, lethargy, sleepiness, and general weakness.

❏ **How Dong Quai Can Help:** Dong quai has long been prescribed by doctors of Chinese medicine as a tonic. Clinical tests have shown that dong quai's mild energizing effect is due to coumarins, a group of active ingredients that stimulate the central nervous system.

❏ **Dosages:** During periodic times of fatigue, enjoy one to three cups of dong quai tea. Dong quai tea can also be used daily to help combat long-term fatigue. However, if you suffer from unexplained fatigue, you may want to consult your physician about possible causes.

BLOOD BUILDER

One of the most common causes of fatigue in women of child bearing years is anemia. Anemia, also called iron-deficiency anemia, occurs when there is not enough iron in the body. Without the proper amount of this mineral, the body cannot produce adequate amounts of hemoglobin. Why does this matter? Hemoglobin is responsible for carrying tissue-nourishing oxygen from the lungs to every part of the body. Without oxygen, the body cannot function properly. A low-iron diet, heavy monthly menstrual flow, pregnancy, recent blood loss (perhaps due to childbirth), and poor iron absorption by the body can all lead to anemia. Signs can be so mild they often go unnoticed: Greater-than-usual fatigue or slight pallor are common symptoms. To treat anemia, doctors of Chinese medicine have long prescribed dong quai, which is known as a blood tonic to them. Modern research supports this claim: Several studies have shown that dong quai contains high levels of blood-building iron.

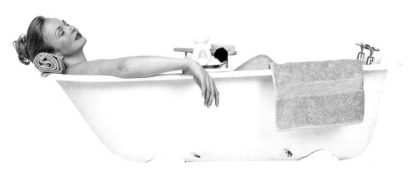

CONDITIONS AND DOSES

DYSMENORRHEA

❏ **Symptoms:** Mild to moderate pain during menstruation is normal and occurs when the uterus contracts to shed its temporary lining. However, sometimes the uterus contracts more than necessary, causing extreme pain. This condition is called dysmenorrhea. It is believed to be caused by excessive levels of prostaglandins. The primary symptom is strong to severe pain in the lower abdomen during menstruation; this pain may radiate to the hips, buttocks, or thighs. Other signs include diarrhea, dizziness, excessive perspiration, fatigue, nausea, and vomiting.

❏ **How Dong Quai Can Help:** Dong quai is an ideal menstrual aid, thanks to a group of active ingredients collectively known as coumarins. It is these ingredients, which boast antispasmodic powers, that relax cramped uterine muscles. The herb also has analgesic powers that deaden severe uterine pain. Furthermore, the herb's mild sedating effects help calm the fear and anxiety that dysmenorrhea often causes. **Note:** Painful periods are not always dysmenorrhea. In some cases they signal an underlying disease, such as endometriosis. If you suffer from painful periods, please see your physician to rule out any existing illness.

❏ **Dosages:** At the first sign of symptoms, enjoy 1 or 2 cups of dong quai tea. For stronger relief, take one 200-mg capsule three times a day; or 1/4 teaspoon of liquid extract three times a day; or 1/2 teaspoon of tincture three times a day. A relaxing dong quai bath is also helpful: To a warm bath, add 1/2 teaspoon of liquid extract or essential oil; or 1 teaspoon of tincture; or 1/2 cup of dried herb.

PREGNANCY CARE

Dong quai is well known for its antispasmodic abilities. The herb has the reverse effect, however, on pregnant individuals, on whom it acts as a uterine stimulant. This means that the herb promotes contractions, making it dangerous for pregnant women. That said, doctors of Chinese medicine regularly prescribe dong quai tea to sip during labor. The herb helps strengthen the contractions that expel the baby from the uterus. Immediately following childbirth, it is a Chinese tradition to serve the new mother a bowl of dong quai soup to deaden pain (dong quai has an analgesic effect) and promote the uterine contractions needed to help the uterus return to its prepregnancy state. Before trying this yourself, please consult a knowledgeable physician.

CONDITIONS AND DOSES

MENOPAUSE

❏ **Symptoms:** Menopause is not an illness but a natural condition that occurs when the ovaries no longer produce enough estrogen to stimulate the lining of the uterus and vagina sufficiently. Simply put, menopause is when women no longer menstruate or get pregnant. It generally occurs somewhere between the ages of 40 and 60. One of the most famous signs of menopause is the hot flash, a sudden reddening of the face accompanied by a feeling of intense warmth. Other common symptoms include depressed mood, fluid retention, headache, insomnia, irritability, nervousness, night sweats, painful intercourse, rapid heartbeat, susceptibility to bladder problems, thinning of vaginal tissues, vaginal dryness, and weight gain. It should be noted that some women experience few symptoms, while still others encounter none at all.

❏ **How Dong Quai Can Help:** A traditional "remedy" for menopause is hormone replacement therapy. This optional treatment uses synthetic hormones to elevate progesterone and estrogen to their premenopausal levels. Dong quai is helpful regardless of whether one undergoes or forgoes hormone replacement therapy. The coumarins in dong quai boast several actions helpful to menopausal symptoms: analgesic action to deaden headaches; antimicrobial action to prevent bladder infections; diuretic action to counteract fluid retention; and sedating action to alleviate insomnia, irritability, and nervousness. Dong quai contains large amounts of vitamin E, which, research has shown, helps diminish hot flashes and vaginal dryness.

❒ **Dosages:** One 200-mg capsule three times a day; or 1/4 teaspoon of liquid extract three times a day; or 1/2 teaspoon of tincture three times a day. With your physician's recommendation, the same dosage can be taken as a complement to hormone replacement therapy.

A NATURAL LAXATIVE
A lack of fiber in the diet, not enough water, and irregular bathroom habits can all lead to constipation. Instead of relying on a chemical laxative, there are natural remedies that are not only gentler, but safer. Bran, fibrous foods, psyllium, and water are natural laxative options that make the stool softer, bulkier, and easier to pass. Dong quai offers another kind of help. For centuries, herbalists and doctors of Chinese medicine have prescribed dong quai tea for constipation. The herb relaxes the muscles of the large intestine, allowing hard, dry stools to pass through.

CONDITIONS AND DOSES

OLIGOMENORRHEA

❒ **Symptoms:** Oligomenorrhea is the medical word for infrequent periods. The word is derived from three Greek words: *oligo*, meaning "few," *men*, which means "month," and *rhoia*, the word for "flow." The primary symptom of oligomenorrhea is less than 11 menstrual periods a year. Infrequent periods are especially common in individuals who suffer from a hormonal imbalance, particularly individuals who have recently stopped taking oral birth control pills or are approaching menopause. However, an imbalance can occur for no apparent reason. **Note:** Because infrequent periods can also be a symptom of excess androgen production or ovarian cancer, it is important to visit a gynecologist if you suffer from oligomenorrhea.

❒ **How Dong Quai Can Help:** Dong quai has been shown in numerous studies to promote menstrual flow. Exactly how dong quai regulates menstruation is unknown; however, it is thought that the herb's high levels of vitamin E may be responsible. In a recent study at Johns Hopkins University, women with hormonal imbalances were given 800 IU of vitamin E for ten weeks. At the end of the trial, test subjects showed balanced hormone levels and normalized menstrual cycles.

❒ **Dosages:** If oligomenorrhea is unexplainable, or caused by a recent discontinuation of oral birth control pills, take one 200-mg capsule three times a day; or 1/4 teaspoon of liquid extract three times a day; or 1/2 teaspoon of tincture three times a day. Discontinue use once regular menstruation occurs.

FERTILITY AID?

Infertility is defined as the inability to conceive after a full year of unprotected intercourse. The problem can lie with the male (up to 40 percent of all cases) or female (up to 60 percent of all cases). Although medical measures—fertility drugs, in vitro fertilization, donor eggs or sperm—can increase the chance of conceiving, medical intervention is costly, physically invasive, and time-consuming. The alternative? Many herbalists claim that dong quai has helped women become pregnant in the presence of unexplained infertility. Indeed, the herb has historically been used by women in China, Korea, and Japan to promote fertility. But does that mean dong quai can make an infertile person fertile? Unfortunately, no large-scale study has been done on the subject. Right now, the medical establishment views dong quai's fertility ability as anecdotal.

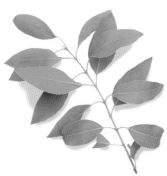

CONDITIONS AND DOSES

PREMENSTRUAL SYNDROME

❐ **Symptoms:** Premenstrual syndrome, popularly known as PMS, is a predictable pattern of physical and emotional changes that occur in some women just before menstruation. Symptoms range from barely noticeable to extreme and can include abdominal swelling, anxiety, bloating, breast soreness, clumsiness, depressed mood, difficulty concentrating, fatigue, fluid retention, headaches, irritability, lethargy, skin eruptions, sleep disturbances, swollen hands and feet, and weight gain.

❐ **How Dong Quai Can Help:** Dong quai is a popular remedy for PMS, thanks to the herb's diuretic qualities, which reduce the swelling, breast soreness, and fluid retention associated with PMS. Furthermore, the herb's analgesic powers relieve headache pain. Dong quai also boasts sedating powers that fight insomnia and irritability; conversely, the herb is also a mild central nervous system stimulant and has a slight energizing effect.

❐ **Dosages:** Two weeks before your period, enjoy 1 or 2 cups of dong quai tea a day. For stronger relief, take one 200-mg capsule three times a day; or 1/4 teaspoon of liquid extract three times a day; or 1/2 teaspoon of tincture three times a day. A relaxing dong quai bath is also helpful: To a warm bath, add 1/2 teaspoon of liquid extract or essential oil; or 1 teaspoon of tincture; or 1/2 cup of dried herb. Discontinue dong quai use on the second day of menstruation. Can be used monthly.

ABOUT PMS

✳ Studies have shown that women who regularly consume three or more cups of coffee daily are four times as likely to have severe PMS as women who drink little or no coffee.

✳ A significant number of PMS sufferers also have some type of thyroid dysfunction.

✳ Recent research suggests that some women who suffer from PMS may be deficient in melatonin. A hormone that regulates the body's biological clock, melatonin is secreted at night by the pineal gland.

✳ In Japan, women suffering from the effects of PMS drink kombuchu tea. This energizing beverage is high in antioxidants and immune-boosting phytochemicals.

✳ Many gynecologists recommend oral contraceptives for women with PMS. Oral contraceptives lessen PMS symptoms by "tricking" the body into believing it is pregnant.

CONDITIONS AND DOSES

RESPIRATORY ALLERGIES

❒ **Symptoms:** A respiratory allergy feels similar to a cold—only with more itchiness. The condition is an immune-system response to a specific airborne allergen, usually animal dander, dust, mold, or pollen. When the allergen is inhaled, an allergic person produces antibodies, which react with the offending substance and prompt the release of histamine. This histamine causes the linings of the nose, sinuses, eyelids, and eyes to become inflamed, producing a variety of symptoms that can include coughing, frequent sneezing, itchiness at the roof of the mouth, itchy eyes, itchy nose, itchy throat, runny nose, stuffy nose, and watery eyes. Interestingly, when a person is allergic to pollen, the allergy is sometimes called hay fever—even though allergies to airborne dander, dust, and mold produce identical symptoms.

❒ **How Dong Quai Can Help:** Studies have shown that dong quai can suppress mild allergic symptoms by altering immune-system reactions. It does this by inhibiting IgE titers, substances that promote immune-system reactions.

❒ **Dosages:** For individuals who are in frequent contact with their "trigger allergen," dong quai can be a preventative when taken as one 200-mg capsule three times a day; or 1/4 teaspoon of liquid extract three times a day; or 1/2 teaspoon of tincture three times a day. For individuals whose contact with their allergen is less frequent, two 200-mg capsules, or 1/2 teaspoon of liquid extract, or 1 teaspoon of tincture can be taken an hour before anticipated contact or immediately upon contact.

DONG QUAI—ON PINS AND NEEDLES

Osteoarthritis, known more popularly as arthritis, is one of the most common disorders known to humans, affecting up to 80 percent of all individuals over the age of 60. Caused by simple wear and tear on a joint, arthritis is considered a degenerative disease. Symptoms include mild to moderately severe pain in a joint during or after use, discomfort in a joint during a weather change, swelling in an affected joint, and loss of flexibility in the joint. Doctors of Chinese medicine treat osteoarthritis with acupuncture, a healing system that uses fine-tipped needles inserted into acupoints to stimulate self-healing. Due to the herb's analgesic properties, many practitioners first dip acupuncture needles into dong quai tea or tincture before inserting them. When used with acupuncture, dong quai is said to deaden a patient's joint pain for two or three days following treatment.

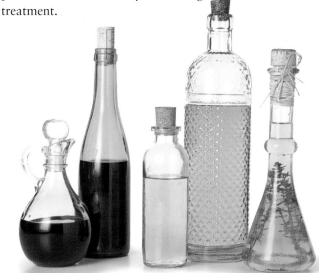

CONDITIONS AND DOSES

STREP THROAT

❏ **Symptoms:** Strep throat is caused by the streptococcus bacteria. In addition to a sore throat, symptoms include difficulty swallowing, swollen lymph nodes, and sometimes a mild fever.

❏ **How Dong Quai Can Help:** Dong quai contains a group of components known as coumarins, which have been shown to kill streptococcus bacteria. The herb also has mild immune system-stimulating powers to help the body fight off infection. Finally, dong quai's analgesic effect slightly deadens pain.

❏ **Dosages:** Gargle three times a day with dong quai tea or dong quai decoction; or take one teaspoon of dong quai syrup, three times a day. In addition, take one 200-mg capsule three times a day; or 1/4 teaspoon of liquid extract three times a day; or 1/2 teaspoon of tincture, three times a day.

GASTROINTESTINAL UPSETS

In Germany, dong quai is referred to as *Angelica sinensis* and is listed in the Commission E monographs as a treatment for flatulence and stomachaches. The herb is a carminative, meaning that it helps the body expel trapped gas. Moreover, dong quai has antispasmodic effects to relax contracting stomach muscles, and it is a well-known gentle analgesic.

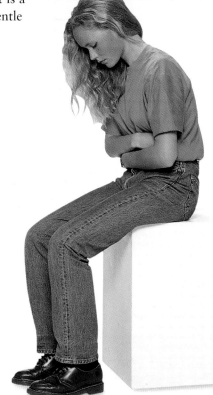

GROW IT YOURSELF

Dong quai may have its roots in the mountains of China, Korea, and Japan, but that hasn't stopped American gardeners from planting it as an ornamental perennial. A slightly slow-growing plant, the herb boasts purplish stems and attractive umbrella-shaped clusters of white flowers. The root, or rhizome as it is also called, is the medicinal and edible part of the plant and can reach lengths of 20 to almost 40 inches.

ANGELICA SINENSIS

The root acts as a blood tonic.

• **Size.** Three to four feet high; can reach heights of seven feet.

• **Native Habitat.** Mountainous areas and high-elevation meadows and streambeds of China, Korea, and Japan.

• **Cultivation.** Prefers rich, moist, well-drained soils and is partial to full sun. Direct-seed during fall, barely covering seeds with soil. Thin to 18 inches apart. Water sparingly and do not prune or fertilize plants. They will flower between May and August. While dong quai roots are harvestable in their first summer, it is better to wait until their third year to harvest.

• **Hint:** Dong quai seeds germinate best in moderately cool to cool temperatures.

GATHERING YOUR OWN

Hunting wild herbs is a satisfying introduction to herbal therapy—but when done thoughtlessly, it can cause plant extinction. In fact, today's increased interest in wild herb gathering has left many indigenous plants extinct; echinacea, ginger, ginseng, goldenseal, sweet grass, and wild carrot are now nearly impossible to find in their native habitats. True, because dong quai does not grow wild in the United States, it is one herb that can't be gathered. But to help protect other native medicinal herbs, ask yourself the following questions before gathering:

✔ Is this plant endangered? If so, it may be illegal in your state to gather it.

✔ Do I need to take this herb from the wild or can I purchase it or grow it myself?

✔ Am I gathering for personal use only and not for commercial use?
Note: Gathering wild plants for commercial use is illegal in many states.

✔ Do I know the plant's mode of reproduction? When gathering a plant that reproduces from seeds, random flowers must be left on each plant in order to generate more seed. When gathering an herb that reproduces from underground rhizomes, plants should be thinned evenly, leaving no discernible "bald patches."

✔ What will I be using this herb for and exactly how much of it do I need?

✔ Are the plants growing in sprayed areas, such as farmland sprayed with pesticides or marshes sprayed for mosquito control?

✔ Can I leave behind enough healthy plants for the local animal population?

✔ Can I leave behind enough healthy plants that can reproduce?

DO-IT-YOURSELF REMEDIES

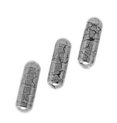

* **Capsule:** Make your own herb supplements by purchasing gelatin or vegetable-gelatin capsules at your local health food store and packing each individual capsule with 200 mg of dried, powdered dong quai root.

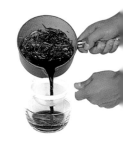

* **Decoction:** Because dong quai root is less permeable than the aerial parts of the plant, simmering the root in boiling water helps extract a greater percentage of its medicinal constituents. To make a decoction, place 25 grams of chopped dried root or 75 grams of chopped fresh root in a nonreactive saucepan. Cover with 750 ml of cold water, place a lid on the saucepan, and boil until the liquid reduces to 500 ml—this usually takes from 20 to 40 minutes. Strain the liquid, and use warm or allow to cool.

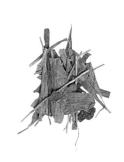

* **Drying:** Wash, thoroughly dry, and chop fresh dong quai root into small pieces. Lay the chopped root on trays in a dry, well-ventilated, nonsunny area of your home or place in an extremely low oven, making sure air is continually circulating around the herbs. Or you can use a dehydrator. Drying will take between five and ten days. When drying herbs either in a warm room or an oven, the temperature should be kept between 70o to 90o F. Store dried root in a dark, airtight, nonporous container.

✳ **Fomentation:** Fomentations are essentially gauze or surgical bandages that are soaked in freshly made herbal tea. The hot cloth is then laid directly on the affected area.

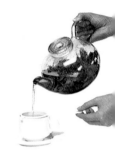

✳ **Infused Oil Made With Fresh or Dried Root:** Infused oils boast the fat-soluble active principles of whatever medicinal plant or herb was used to make them. To make dong quai oil, place 200 grams of dried dong quai root in a nonreactive saucepan and cover with 500 ml of almond or olive oil. Simmer over very low heat for three hours. Allow mixture to cool. Strain the oil and store it in a dark, airtight container for up to two years. Can be ingested or used externally.

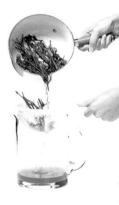

✳ **Liquid Extract.** Also known as extract. To make dong quai extract, macerate 100 to 200 grams of dried dong quai root, or 300 to 500 grams of fresh dong quai root. Place the herb in a jar and pour in 335 ml vodka (37 proof or higher) and 165 ml water. Place the lid on the jar and store in a dark area for four to eight weeks. Shake the mixture daily. When ready, strain the mixture, pressing all remaining liquid from the dong quai root. Place liquid in a nonreactive saucepan and simmer over medium heat for 20 to 40 minutes until the liquid has been reduced by a third. This process burns off the alcohol, leaving the medicinal liquid behind. Allow liquid to cool and decant into several dropper bottles or a clean glass bottle. Will keep up to two years. Shake before using.

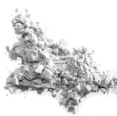

DO-IT-YOURSELF REMEDIES

❋ **Ointment:** Also called a salve, herbal ointment is easy to make at home. To create your own dong quai ointment for muscle aches, mix 1 to 2 parts beeswax or soft paraffin wax, 7 parts cocoa butter, and 3 parts powdered dong quai root, in a nonreactive saucepan. Cook the mixture for one to two hours on a low setting. Let cool and then package in an airtight container. Rub into aching muscle up to three times a day.

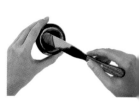

❋ **Poultice:** Fresh herbs can be applied directly to bites and rashes when fashioned into a poultice. To make a dong quai poultice, chop fresh or dried root. Boil in a small amount of water for 5 minutes (or use a microwave). Squeeze out any excess liquid from the boiled herb (reserve liquid). Lay the dong quai directly on the affected area and cover with a warm moist towel. Leave in place for up to 30 minutes. The reserved liquid can be rewarmed and used to reheat the towel.

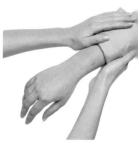

❋ **Syrup:** Dong quai has a bittersweet taste that may not be palatable to some individuals. Syrup delivers the herb's medicinal benefits in an easy-to-swallow (and throat-soothing) base. To make, mix 7 parts dong quai tea or decoction in a non-reactive saucepan with 10 parts sugar. Cook the mixture over low heat until it has formed a thick, syrupy, consistency.

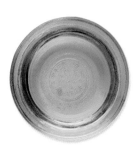

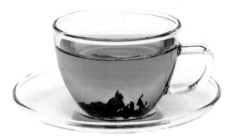

❋ **Tea:** Also known as an infusion, tea is an easy and common way to ingest an herb. To make dong quai tea, steep 1 teaspoon dried root or 1 tablespoon fresh leaves for 5 minutes in 1 cup of boiling water. You may add fructose, sugar, or honey to sweeten.

❋ **Tinctures:** Though not as potent as liquid extracts, tinctures are minimally processed, making them a favorite remedy among many herbalists. To make your own dong quai tincture, place 100 to 200 grams of dried dong quai root, or 300 to 500 grams of fresh dong quai root, in a large jar and cover with 500 ml vodka (37 proof or higher). Place the lid on the jar and store in a dark area for four to six weeks. Shake the bottle daily. When ready to use, strain the mixture, pressing all remaining liquid from the dong quai root. Decant into several dropper bottles or a clean glass bottle. Will keep for up to two years. Shake before using.

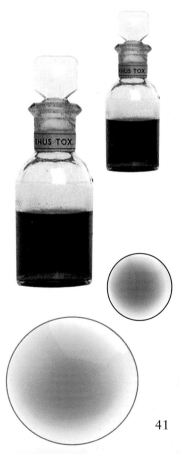

ALTERNATIVE HEALTH STRATEGIES

Herbs, vitamins, minerals—sure these contribute to good health. But creating general well-being involves more than simply taking supplements. Good health has to do with various quality-of-life issues that can aggravate or cause stress, thus harming health. Here are some additional ways to help keep yourself well.

Improve Your Eating Habits
Here are the five main eating strategies people follow; consider finding the most healthful one that works with your lifestyle.

- OMNIVOROUS
- PISCATORIAL
- MACROBIOTIC
- VEGAN
- VEGETARIAN

Get More Exercise
Whether it's walking or weightlifting, any type of exercise can help you feel better. Try any of these types:

- STRETCHING
- AEROBICS
- STRENGTH TRAINING

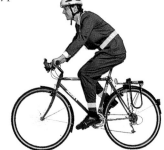

Simple Ways To Ease Stress

In addition to exercise and healthy eating, here are some more techniques–old and new–for easing stress and increasing relaxation.

- GET ENOUGH SLEEP
- MEDITATE REGULARLY
- GIVE UP JUNK FOOD
- ADOPT A PET
- SURROUND YOURSELF WITH SUPPORTIVE PEOPLE
- LIMIT YOUR EXPOSURE TO CHEMICALS
- TAKE YOUR VITAMINS
- ENJOY YOURSELF

ONE-MINUTE STRESS REDUCER

Stress is one of the top health hazards we face today. Unfortunately, it's impossible to go through life without the irritations that make us tense. Fortunately, there *is* something you can do to minimize their power to aggravate you. It's called deep breathing, and it can be done anywhere and anytime you need to calm and center yourself. Here's how:

1. Inhale deeply through your nose.
2. Hold your breath for up to three seconds, then exhale your breath through your mouth.
3. Continue as needed.

Deep breathing pulls a person's attention away from a given stressor and refocuses it on his or her breath. This type of breathing is not only comforting (thanks to its rhythmic quality), but also has been shown to lower rapid pulse and shallow respiration—two temporary symptoms of stress.

EATING SMART

A balanced diet is the foundation of good health. For proof, just read the numerous medical studies that link healthful eating with disease prevention and disease reversal. These same studies connect high fat intake, high sodium consumption, and diets with too much protein to numerous illnesses, including cancer, cardiovascular diseases, diverticular diseases, hypertension, and heart disease. But what exactly is a balanced diet? Generally speaking, it is a diet comprised of carbohydrates, dietary fiber, fat, protein, water, 13 vitamins, and 20 minerals. More specifically, it is a diet built around a wide variety of fruits, legumes, whole grains and vegetables. Alcohol, animal protein, high-fat foods, high-sodium foods, highly sugared foods, sodas, and processed foods are consumed sparingly, if at all.

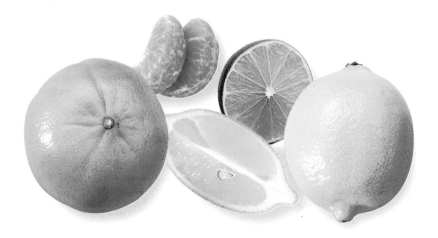

OMNIVOROUS

❑ **On The Menu:** Plant-based foods, dairy products, eggs, fish, seafood, red meats, organ meats, poultry.

❑ **Foods That Are Avoided:** None. Everything is fair game.

❑ **How Healthy Is It?** It depends. Someone who eats eggs, poultry, or meat every day, chooses refined snacks over whole foods, and gets only one or two daily servings of fruits and vegetables will not be as healthy as a person who limits meat (the general dietary term for any "flesh foods," including poultry and fish) to two or three times a week, chooses water over soft drinks, and gets the recommended five or more daily servings of fruits and vegetables. Complaints about traditional omnivorous diets revolve around the diet's high levels of cholesterol and saturated fat (found in animal-based foods), which increase the risk of cancer, diabetes, heart disease, and obesity.

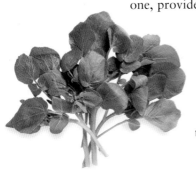

However, an omnivorous diet can be healthful one, provided thoughtful choices are made. To keep cholesterol and saturated fat to a minimum and nutrients to a maximum, eat five or more daily servings of fruits and vegetables, choose whole grains over refined grains, enjoy daily legume or soyfood protein sources, and limit the use of animal foods.

EATING SMART

MACROBIOTIC

❏ **On The Menu:** Plant-based foods, fish, very limited amounts of salt.

❏ **Foods That Are Avoided:** Dairy products, eggs, foods with artificial ingredients, hot spices, mass-produced foods, organ meats, peppers, potatoes, poultry, red meats, shellfish, warm drinks, refined foods.

❏ **How Healthy Is It?** Macrobiotics is based on a system created in the early 1900s by Japanese philosopher George Ohsawa. The diet consists of 50 percent whole grains, 20 to 30 percent vegetables, and 5 to 10 percent beans, sea vegetables, and soy foods. The remainder of the diet is composed of white-meat fish, fruits, and nuts. The diet's low amounts of saturated fat, absence of processed foods, and emphasis on high-fiber foods such as whole grains and vegetables, may promote cardiovascular health. Because soy and sea vegetables contain cancer-fighting compounds, a macrobiotic diet is often recommended to help treat cancer. However, critics worry that the diet's limited variety of food can leave followers lacking in certain vitamins and important cancer-fighting phytonutrients.

PISCATORIAL

❏ **On The Menu:** Plant-based foods, dairy products, eggs, fish, seafood.

❏ **Foods That Are Avoided:** Red meats, organ meats, poultry.

❏ **How Healthy Is It?** Like an omnivorous diet, a piscatorial diet is as healthy as a person makes it. Individuals who eat high-fat and highly processed foods fail to get the recommended daily number of vegetables and fruits, and eschew whole grains for processed grains will not enjoy optimum health. That said, individuals who are conscientious about eating a balanced, varied diet, and who limit fish and seafood intake to two or three times per week, can expect a lower risk of heart disease. Since many oily fish contain omega-3 fatty acids, eating them in moderation has been found to help lower blood cholesterol. Be aware, however, that oily saltwater fish, such as shark, swordfish and tuna, have been found to carry mercury in their tissues; many health authorities recommend eating these varieties no more than once or twice a week. Also, due to overfishing, many fish species are now threatened, including bluefin tuna, Pacific perch, Chilean sea bass, Chinook salmon, and swordfish. For additional information on endangered fish, visit the University of Michigan's Endangered Species Update at www.umich.edu/~esuupdate, or the Fish and Wildlife Information Exchange at http://fwie.fe.vt.edu.

EATING SMART

VEGAN

❏ **On The Menu:** Plant-based foods.

❏ **Foods That Are Avoided:** Dairy, eggs, fish, seafood, red meats, organ meats, poultry. Also avoided are foods made by animals or processed with animal parts, such as gelatin, honey, marshmallows made with animal gelatin, white sugar processed with bone char.

❏ **How Healthy Is It?** A vegan (pronounced VEE-gun) diet can be extremely healthful. Like the vegetarian diet, a vegan diet has been shown by numerous studies to lower blood pressure and prevent heart disease. In addition, the high fiber intake cuts the risk of diverticular disease and colon cancer. Yet because vegans do not eat dairy products or eggs, they must be more conscientious than vegetarians about eating plant foods with vitamin B_{12} and vitamin D or taking supplements of these nutrients.

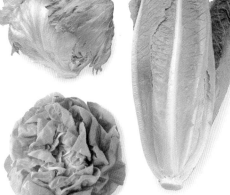

VEGETARIAN

❐ **On The Menu:** Plant-based foods, dairy, eggs.

❐ **Foods That Are Avoided:** Fish, gelatin, seafood, red meats, organ meats, poultry.

❐ **How Healthy Is It?** A vegetarian diet can be very healthful when done right. Fortunately, this isn't hard. Dietary science has debunked theories of "protein combining" popular in the 1960s and 1970s, leaving today's vegetarians to worry only about eating a wide variety of whole foods, including beans, fruits, grains, low-fat dairy products, nuts, soy foods, and vegetables. A varied daily diet insures enough protein, calcium, and other nutrients for vegetarians of all ages, including children, pregnant individuals, and the elderly. A well-chosen vegetarian eating plan has been shown by numerous studies to lower blood pressure, decrease the risk of breast cancer, and prevent heart disease. In addition, the diet's high fiber levels cut the risk of diverticular disease and colon cancer.

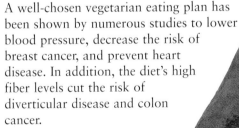

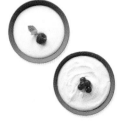

HERB GLOSSARY

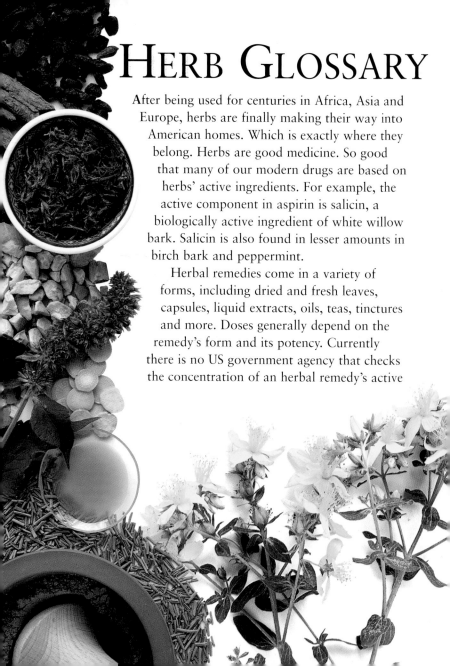

After being used for centuries in Africa, Asia and Europe, herbs are finally making their way into American homes. Which is exactly where they belong. Herbs are good medicine. So good that many of our modern drugs are based on herbs' active ingredients. For example, the active component in aspirin is salicin, a biologically active ingredient of white willow bark. Salicin is also found in lesser amounts in birch bark and peppermint.

Herbal remedies come in a variety of forms, including dried and fresh leaves, capsules, liquid extracts, oils, teas, tinctures and more. Doses generally depend on the remedy's form and its potency. Currently there is no US government agency that checks the concentration of an herbal remedy's active

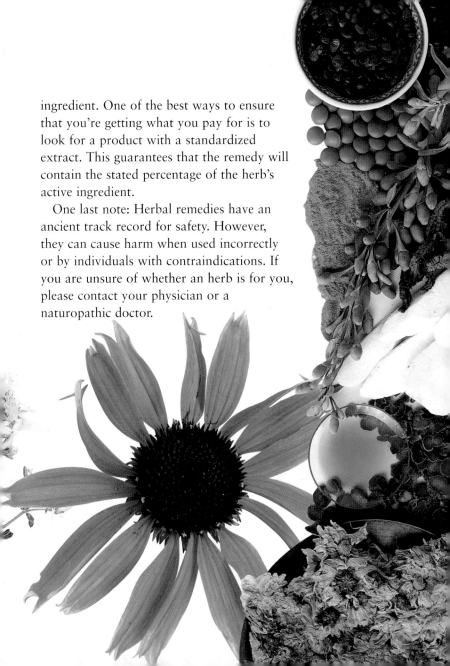

ingredient. One of the best ways to ensure that you're getting what you pay for is to look for a product with a standardized extract. This guarantees that the remedy will contain the stated percentage of the herb's active ingredient.

One last note: Herbal remedies have an ancient track record for safety. However, they can cause harm when used incorrectly or by individuals with contraindications. If you are unsure of whether an herb is for you, please contact your physician or a naturopathic doctor.

ALOE

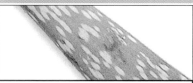

Properties: Analgesic, antibacterial, antifungal, anti-inflammatory, anti-itch, antiseptic, circulatory stimulant, digestive aid, immune-system stimulant, laxative.
Target Ailments: Acne, bruises, burns, constipation, cuts, insect bites, digestive disorders, rashes, ulcers, wounds.
Available Forms: Capsule, fresh leaves, gel, juice, liquid extract.
Possible Side Effects: When taken internally, aloe can cause severe cramping in some individuals.
Precautions: Pregnant women should not ingest aloe; It can stimulate uterine contractions.

CALENDULA

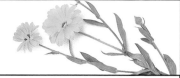

Properties: Antibacterial, anti-inflammatory, antiseptic, antispasmodic, promotes sweating, sedative.
Target Ailments: Burns, cuts, fungal infections, gallbladder conditions, hepatitis, indigestion, irregular menstruation, insect bites, menstrual cramps, mouth sores, skin rashes, ulcers, wounds.
Available Forms: Capsule, dried herb, fresh herb, liquid extract, lotion, oil, ointment, tincture.
Possible Side Effects: None expected.
Precautions: Calendula is related to ragweed. Individuals allergic to ragweed should consult a physician before using calendula.

ASTRAGALUS

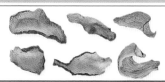

Properties: Antibacterial, anti-inflammatory, antioxidant, antiviral, diuretic, immune-system stimulant.
Target Ailments: Cancer, colds, appetite loss, diarrhea, fatigue, flu, heart conditions, HIV, viral infections.
Available Forms: Capsule, dried herb, fresh herb, liquid extract, tea, tincture.
Possible Side Effects: None expected.
Precautions: Astragalus should be used as a companion therapy to—not a replacement for—traditional cancer and HIV therapies.

CHAMOMILE

Properties: Antibacterial, anti-inflammatory, antiseptic, antispasmodic, carminative, digestive aid, fever reducer, sedative.
Target Ailments: Gingivitis, hemorrhoids, insomnia, indigestion, intestinal gas, menstrual cramps, nausea, nervousness, stomachaches, sunburns, tension, ulcers, varicose veins.
Available Forms: Capsule, dried herb, fresh herb, liquid extract, lotion, oil, tea, tincture.
Possible Side Effects: None expected.
Precautions: Because chamomile is related to ragweed, individuals with ragweed allergies should consult a physician before using chamomile.

DONG QUAI

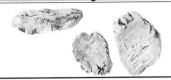

Properties: Antiallergenic, antispasmodic, diuretic, mild laxative, muscle relaxant, vasodilator.
Target Ailments: Abscesses, blurred vision, heart palpitations, irregular menstruation, light-headedness, menstrual pain, pallor, poor circulation.
Available Forms: Capsule, dried herb, liquid extract, tincture.
Possible Side Effects: Can cause photosensitivity in some individuals.
Precautions: Dong quai has abortive abilities; Do not take while pregnant.

FEVERFEW

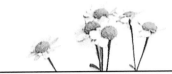

Properties: Anti-inflammatory, fever reducer.
Target Ailments: Arthritis, asthma, dermatitis, menstrual pain, migraines.
Available Forms: Capsule, dried herb, fresh herb, liquid extract, tincture.
Possible Side Effects: Some individuals experience "withdrawal" symptoms after taking feverfew, including fatigue and nervousness.
Precautions: Because it is related to ragweed, individuals with ragweed allergies should consult a physician before using feverfew.

ECHINACEA

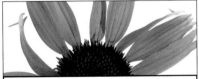

Properties: Antiallergenic, antibacterial, antiseptic, antimicrobial, antiviral, carminative, lymphatic tonic.
Target Ailments: Abscesses, acne, bladder infections, blood poisoning, burns, colds, eczema, food poisoning, flu, insect bites, kidney infections, mononucleosis, respiratory infections, sore throats.
Available Forms: Capsule, dried herb, liquid extract, tea, tincture.
Possible Side Effects: High doses can cause dizziness and nausea.
Precautions: Do not take echinacea for more than four weeks in a row.

GARLIC

Properties: Antibacterial, anticoagulant, antifungal, anti-inflammatory, antiviral, cholesterol reducer, digestive aid, immune-system stimulant, worm-fighting.
Target Ailments: Arteriosclerosis, arthritis, bladder infections, colds, digestive upset, flu, heart conditions, high blood pressure, high blood cholesterol, viral infections.
Available Forms: Capsule, fresh cloves, liquid extract, oil, tincture.
Possible Side Effects: Can cause upset stomach.
Precautions: While garlic is safe taken in culinary doses, individuals on anticoagulant medications should consult their doctors before supplementing their diet with garlic.

GINGER

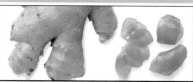

Properties: Antibacterial, anticoagulant, antinausea, antispasmodic, antiviral, carminative, digestive aid, expectorant, immune-system stimulant, muscle relaxant.

Target Ailments: Burns, colds, flu, high blood pressure, high cholesterol, liver conditions, intestinal gas, menstrual cramps, motion sickness, nausea, stomachaches.

Available Forms: Capsule, dried root, tea.

Possible Side Effects: Heartburn.

Precautions: While ginger is safe in culinary doses, individuals who suffer from a blood-clotting disorder or are on anticoagulant medication should consult a physician before supplementing their diet with the herb.

GINSENG

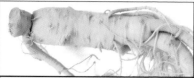

Properties: Antibacterial, antidepressant, immune-system stimulant, stimulant.

Target Ailments: Colds, depression, fatigue, flu, impaired immune system, respiratory conditions, stress.

Available Forms: Capsule, dried root, fresh root, liquid extract, tincture, tea.

Possible Side Effects: Large doses of ginseng can cause breast soreness, headaches or skin rashes in some individuals.

Precautions: Ginseng can aggravate existing heart palpitations or high blood pressure.

GINKGO BILOBA

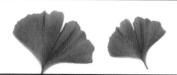

Properties: Antibacterial, anti-inflammatory, antioxidant, circulatory stimulant, vasodilator.

Target Ailments: Clotting disorders, dementia, depression, headaches, hearing loss, Raynaud's syndrome, tinnitus, vascular diseases, vertigo.

Available Forms: Capsule, dry herb, liquid extract, tincture, tea.

Possible Side Effects: Diarrhea, irritability, nausea, restlessness.

Precautions: Do not use ginkgo biloba if you have a blood-clotting disorder like hemophilia or are taking anticoagulant medications.

GOLDENSEAL

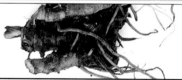

Properties: Antacid, antibacterial, antifungal, anti-inflammatory, antiseptic, astringent, digestive aid, stimulant.

Target Ailments: Canker sores, contact dermatitis, diarrhea, eczema, food poisoning.

Available Forms: Capsule, dry herb, liquid extract, tea, tincture.

Possible Side Effects: In high doses, goldenseal can cause diarrhea and nausea and can irritate the skin, mouth and throat.

Precautions: Because of its high cost, many manufacturers adulterate preparations with less costly herbs, such as barberry, yellow dock or bloodroot, some of which can cause unwanted reactions when taken in high doses.

KAVA

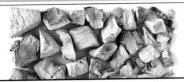

Properties: Antidepressant, antispasmodic, aphrodisiac, diuretic, muscle relaxant, sedative.

Target Ailments: Anxiety, colds, depression, menstrual conditions, muscle cramps, respiratory tract conditions, stress.

Available Forms: Capsule, dried herb, liquid extract, tea, tincture.

Possible Side Effects: Allergic skin reactions, muscle weakness, red eyes, sleepiness.

Precautions: In high doses, kava can impair motor reflexes and cause breathing problems.

MILK THISTLE

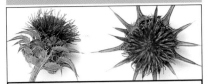

Properties: Anti-inflammatory, antioxidant, digestive aid, immune-system stimulant.

Target Ailments: inflammation of the gallbladder duct, hepatitis, liver conditions, poisoning from ingestion of the death cup mushroom, psoriasis.

Available Forms: Capsule, dried herb, fresh herb, powder, tea, tincture.

Possible Side Effects: Milk thistle can cause mild diarrhea when taken in large doses.

Precautions: If you think you have a liver disorder, seek medical advice before taking this herb.

LAVENDER

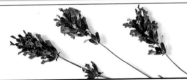

Properties: Antibacterial, antidepressant, antiseptic, antispasmodic, carminative, circulatory stimulant, digestive aid, diuretic, sedative.

Target Ailments: Anxiety, depression, headache, insomnia, intestinal gas, nausea, tension.

Available Forms: Capsule, dried herb, fresh herb, oil, tincture.

Possible Side Effects: Lavender products can cause skin irritation in sensitive individuals.

Precautions: Lavender oil is poisonous when ingested internally.

PARSLEY

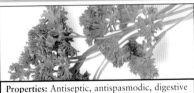

Properties: Antiseptic, antispasmodic, digestive aid, diuretic, laxative, muscle relaxant.

Target Ailments: Colds, congestion, fever, flu, indigestion, irregular menstruation, premenstrual syndrome, stimulating the production of breast milk, stomachaches.

Available Forms: Capsule, dried herb, fresh herb, liquid extract, oil, tea, tincture.

Possible Side Effects: Can cause photosensitivity in some individuals.

Precautions: Parsley should not be ingested in large amounts or used externally during pregnancy; it contains compounds that may stimulate uterine muscles and possibly cause miscarriage.

PEPPERMINT

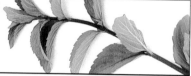

Properties: Antacid, antibacterial, antidepressant, antispasmodic, carminatve, expectorant, muscle relaxant, promotes sweating.
Target Ailments: Anxiety, colds, fever, flu, insomnia, intestinal gas, itching, migraines, morning sickness, motion sickness, nausea.
Available Forms: Capsule, dried herb, fresh herb, lozenge, oil, ointment, tea, tincture.
Possible Side Effects: When applied externally, peppermint products can cause skin reactions in sensitive individuals.
Precautions: If you have a hiatal hernia, talk to your doctor before using peppermint products externally or internally; the oil in the plant can exacerbate symptoms.

SAGE

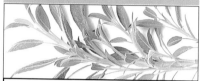

Properties: Antiseptic, anti-inflammatory, antioxidant, antispasmodic, astringent, bile stimulant, carminative, reduces perspiration.
Target Ailments: Excess intestinal gas, insect bites, menopausal night sweats, poor circulation, reduces milk flow at weaning, sore throat, stomachaches, mouth ulcers.
Available Forms: Capsule, dried herb, fresh herb, liquid extract, oil, tincture.
Possible Side Effects: Sage tea may cause inflammation of the lips and/or tongue in some individuals.
Precautions: Do not ingest pure sage oil; it is toxic when taken internally.

ROSEMARY

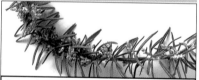

Properties: Antibacterial, antidepressant, anti-inflammatory, antiseptic, carminative, circultory stimulant.
Target Ailments: Bad breath, dandruff, depression, eczema, headaches, indigestion, joint inflammation, mouth and throat infections, muscle pain, psoriasis, rheumatoid arthritis.
Available Forms: Dried herb, fresh herb, ingestible rosemary-flavored oil, oil, ointment, tea, tincture.
Possible Side Effects: Rosemary oil can cause skin inflammation and/or dermatitis.
Precautions: Do not mistake regular rosemary oil for ingestible rosemary-flavored oil.

SAW PALMETTO

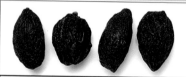

Properties: Antiallergenic, anti-inflammatory, diuretic, immune-boosting.
Target Ailments: Asthma, benign prostatic hyperplasia, bronchitis, colds, cystitis, impotence, male infertility, nasal congestion, sinus conditions, sore throats.
Available Forms: Capsule, dried herb, fresh herb, liquid extract, oil, tea, tincture.
Possible Side Effects: Can cause diarrhea if taken in large doses.
Precautions: Due to its hormonal actions, saw palmetto may interact negatively with prostate medicines or hormonal treatments such as estrogen replacement therapy, possibly canceling out their effectiveness.

ST. JOHN'S WORT

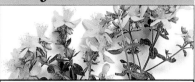

Properties: Analgesic, antibacterial, anti-depressant, anti-inflammatory, antiviral, astringent.
Target Ailments: Attention deficit disorder, anxiety, bacterial infections, burns, carpal tunnel syndrome, depression, HIV, menopause.
Available Forms: Capsule, dried herb, liquid extract, oil, ointment, tea, tincture.
Possible Side Effects: Gastrointestinal upset, headaches, photosensitivity, stiff neck.
Precautions: Avoid foods containing the amino acid tyramine when taking St. John's wort; the interaction of the two can cause an increase in blood pressure. Foods with tyramine include beer, coffee, wine, chocolate and fava beans.

WILD YAM

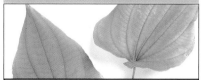

Properties: Analgesic, anti-inflammatory, antispasmodic, expectorant, muscle relaxant, promotes sweating.
Target Ailments: Menopause, menstrual cramps, morning sickness, nausea, rheumatoid arthritis, urinary tract infections.
Available Forms: Capsule, cream, dried root, liquid extract, oil, powder, tincture.
Possible Side Effects: Can cause vomiting in large doses.
Precautions: Individuals who are suffering from a hormone-sensitive cancer, such as breast or uterine cancer, should avoid wild yam. Some experts believe that the herb can encourage the growth of cancer cells.

VALERIAN

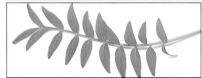

Properties: Analgesic, antibacterial, antispasmodic, carminative, reduces blood pressure, sedative, tranquilizer.
Target Ailments: Brachial spasm, high blood pressure, insomnia, palpitations, menstrual pain, migraines, muscle cramps, nervousness, tension headaches, wounds.
Available Forms: Capsules, dried herb, liquid extract, oil, teas, tincture.
Possible Side Effects: Headaches with prolonged use.
Precautions: Do not take with other sedatives, including alcohol. Do not drive or operate machinery after taking valerian.

YARROW

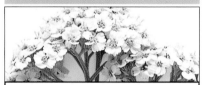

Properties: Antibacterial, anti-inflammatory, antispasmodic, blood coagulator, bile stimulating, immune-system stimulant, promotes sweating, sedative.
Target Ailments: Anxiety, colds and flu, cystitis, digestive disorders, menstrual cramps, minor wounds, nosebleeds, poor circulation, skin rashes.
Available Forms: Dried herb, capsule, liquid extract, oil, tea, tincture.
Possible Side Effects: Diarrhea, skin rash.
Precautions: Yarrow is related to ragweed and can cause an allergic reaction in individuals with ragweed allergies. Do not take if pregnant; it can induce miscarriage.

HERBAL TERMS

You're thumbing through the latest herbal therapy book when you run smack into the word "emmenagogue." Or perhaps you get tangled on "oxytocic." For anyone who's ever been stopped by an unfamiliar alternative medical term, we offer the following list:

Adaptogenic: Increases resistance and resilience to stress. Supports adrenal gland functioning.

Alterative: Blood purifier that improves the condition of the blood, improves digestion, and increases the appetite. Used to treat conditions arising from or causing toxicity.

Analgesic: Herb that relieves pain either by relaxing muscles or reducing pain signals to the brain.

Anthelmintic: Destroys or expels intestinal worms.

Antacid: Neutralizes excess stomach and intestinal acids.

Antiallergenic: Inactivates allergenic substances in the body.

Antibacterial/Antibiotic: Helps the body fight off harmful bacteria.

Antidepressant: Helps maintain emotional stability.

Anticatarrhal: Eliminates or counteracts the formation of mucus.

Anticoagulant: Thins blood and helps prevent blood clots.

Antifungal: Kills infection-causing fungi.

Anti-inflammatory: Reduces swelling of the tissues.

Anti-itch: Deadens itching sensations.

Antimicrobial: Kills a wide range of harmful bacteria, fungi, and viruses.

Antioxidant: Fights harmful oxidation.

Antipyretic/Fever Reducer: Reduces or prevents fever.

Antiseptic: External application prevents bacterial growth on skin.

Antispasmodic: Prevents or relaxes muscle tension.

Antiviral: Helps the body fight invading viruses.

Astringent: Has a constricting or binding effect. Commonly used to treat hemorrhages, secretions and diarrhea.

Blood Coagulant: Thickens blood and aids in clotting.

Carminative: Relieves gas.

Cholagogue: Encourages the flow of bile into the small intestine.

Circulatory Stimulant: Promotes even and efficient blood circulation.

Demulcent: Soothing substance, usually mucilage, taken internally to protect injured or inflamed tissues.

Diaphoretic: Induces sweating.

Diuretic: Increases urine flow.

Emetic: Induces vomiting.

Emmenagogue: Promotes menstruation.

Emollient: Softens, soothes and protects skin.

Expectorant: Assists in expelling mucus from the lungs and throat.

Galactogogue: Increases the secretion of breast milk.

Hemostatic: Stops hemorrhaging and encourages blood coagulation.

Hepatic: Tones and strengthens the liver.

Hypotensive: Lowers abnormally elevated blood pressure.

Immune-System Stimulant: Strengthens immune system so the body can fight off invading organisms.

Laxative: Promotes bowel movements.

Lithotriptic: Helps dissolve urinary and biliary stones.

Muscle Relaxant: Loosens tight muscles and reduces muscle cramping.

Nervine: Calms tension.

Oxytocic: Stimulates uterine contractions.

Rubefacient: Increases blood flow at the surface of the skin.

Sedative: Quiets the nervous system.

Sialagogue/Digestive Aid: Promotes the flow of saliva.

Stimulant: Increases the body's energy.

Tonic: Promotes the functions of body systems.

Vasoconstrictor: Constricts blood vessels, limiting the amount of blood flowing to a particular area.

Vasodilator: Dilates blood vessels, helping to promote blood flow.

Vulnerary: Encourages wound healing by promoting cell growth and repair.

HERBAL ORGANIZATIONS

Where to go for more information:

American Botanical Council
P.O. Box 201660
Austin, TX 78720
512-331-8868
www.herbalgram.org

The American Herbalist Guild
P.O. Box 746555
Arvada, CO 80006
303-423-8800

American Herbalists Guild
Box 1683
Soquel, CA 95073
408-464-2441

Herb Research Foundation
1007 Pearl Street, Suite 200
Boulder, CO 80302
303-449-2265
www.herbs.org

**National Accupuncture and
Oriental Medicine Alliance**
14637 Starr Road SE
Olalla, WA 98359
206-851-6896

**National Institutes of Health
Office of Alternative Medicine**
9000 Rockville Pike
Building 31, Room 5B-37
Mailstop 2182
Bethesda, MD 20892
301-402-2466

The Herb Society of America
9019 Kirtland-Chardon Road
Kirtland, OH 44094
216-256-0514

American College of Sports Medicine
P.O. Box 1440
Indianapolis, IN 46206
317-637-9200

National Health Information Center
P.O. Box 1133
Washington, DC 20013
800-336-4797

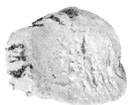
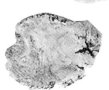
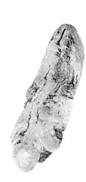

GROWING HERBS

Interested in cultivating herbs yourself?
These sources can supply roots, plants, and/or seeds.

Catoctin Mountain Botanicals
P.O. Box 454
Jefferson, MD 21755
301-473-4351

Companion Plants
7247 N. Coolville Ridge Rd.
Athens, OH 45701
614-593-3092
E-mail: complants@frognet.net

Dry Fork Herb Gardens
R.R.#1 Box 21
Rockport, IL
217-437-5281

Ecofriendly Farms
15488 Barn Rock Rd.
Mendota, VA 24270
540-466-8689

Goodwin Creek Gardens
P.O. Box 83
Williams, OR 97544
541-846-7357

Herbal Exchange
P.O. Box 429
9160 Lentz Rd.
Frazeysburg, OH 43822
614-828-9968

Horizon Herbs
P.O. Box 69
Williams, OR 97544
541-846-6233
www.chatlink.com/~herbseed
E-mail: herbseed@chatlink.com

Johnny's Seeds
Rt. 1 Box 2580
Foss Hill Rd.
Albion, ME 04910
207-437-9294
www.johnnyseeds.com

Mountain Traditions
H.C. 68, Box 193
Big Creek, KY 40914
606-598-6904

Nature's Cathedral
Rt. 1 Box 120
Blairstown, IA 52209
319-454-6959

Prairie Moon Nursery
Rt. 3, Box 163
Winona, MN 55987
507-452-1362

Wilcox Natural Products
P.O. Box 391
755 George Wilson Rd.
Boone, NC 28607
828-264-3615
www.goldenseal.com

Wild Wonderful Farm, Inc.
P.O. Box 256
Franklin, WV 26268
212-736-1467

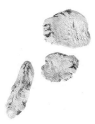

INDEX

ABOUT THE AUTHOR

Stephanie Pedersen is a writer and editor who specializes in the area of health. Her articles have appeared in numerous publications, including *American Woman, Sassy, Teen, Weight Watchers* and *Woman's World*. She has also co-written *What Your Cat is Trying to Tell You: A Head-to-Tail Guide to Your Cat's Symptoms and Their Solutions* and *What Your Dog is Trying to Tell You: A Head-to-Tail Guide to Your Dog's Symptoms and Their Solutions*, both published by St. Martin's Press. She currently resides in New York City.

Picture Credits: Steve Gorton, David Murray, Dave King, Martin Norris, Philip Gatward, Andy Crawford, Philip Dowell, Clive Streeter, Peter Chadwick, Tim Ridley, Andrew Whittack, Martin Cameron

DORLING KINDERSLEY PUBLISHING, INC.
www.dk.com

Published in the United States by
Dorling Kindersley Publishing, Inc.
95 Madison Avenue • New York, New York 10016

Copyright © 2000 by Dorling Kindersley Publishing, Inc.

Editorial Director: LaVonne Carlson
Editors: Nancy Burke, Barbara Minton, Connie Robinson
Designer: Carol Wells
Cover Designer: Gus Yoo

Pedersen, Stephanie.
    Dong Quai : women's wonder drug / by Stephanie Pedersen.
    p.cm. -- (Natural care library)
    Includes index.
    ISBN 0-7894-5193-X (pbk. : alk. paper)
    1. Angelica--Therapeutic use. 2. Women--Diseases--Alternative treatment. 3. Menopause--Alternative treatment. I. Title.
II. Series.
RS165A5P43 2000
615'. 323849--dc21
99-43067

First American Edition   10 9 8 7 6 5 4 3 2 1